Comfort Zones My Arse!

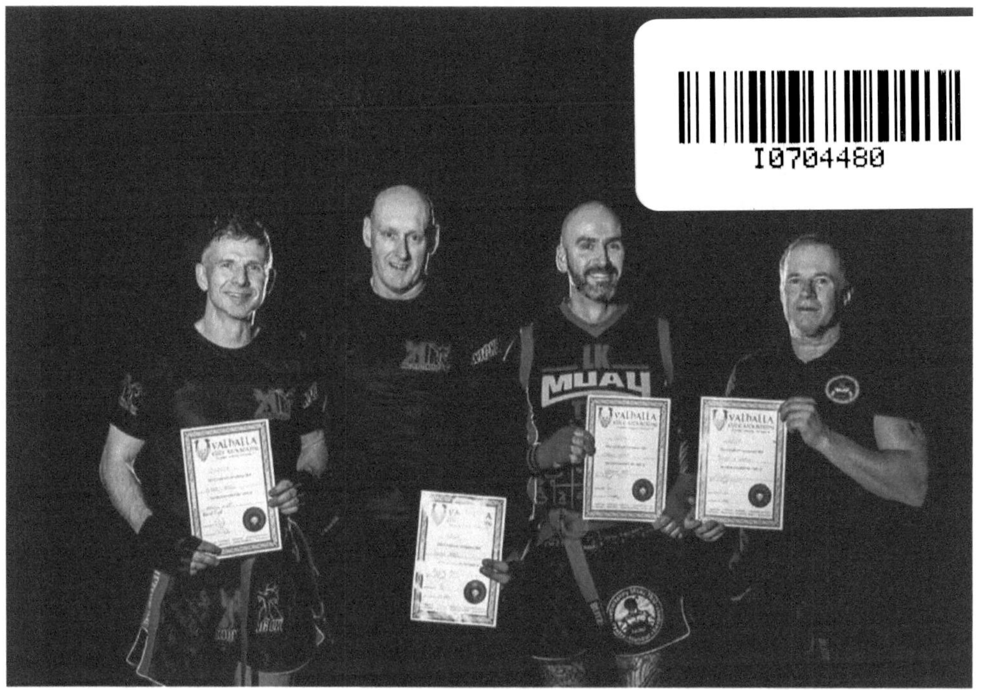

Forward:

This is dedicated to my wife, Carmel and my three daughters, Chloe, Serena and Katie. They walked every step of the way to what you are about to read. In hind-sight was it a selfish thing to do? Maybe. But they encouraged and pushed me to achieve my ambition and reach my goal. To my coach and good friend Tommy 'The Ghost' McCafferty for everything he has done along the way (including a simple gesture that got me back on-track). To my own family and Carmel's family for their unwavering support throughout this journey and to my close friends and work colleagues who knew what achieving my goal meant to me – Thank you!

This is also dedicated to every single person who has, even the smallest bit of self-doubt when it comes to managing their Fitness Health and Wellbeing that "If I can do it…So can you"!

"It's not the size of the dog in the fight but the size of the fight in the dog"

Introduction

"Sparring against a twice ISKA Kickboxing World Champion"!

"Sparring against European and Irish Kickboxing Champions"!

"Five hundred press-ups and sit-ups a day"!

"Fitting in five hours training a day whilst working full time"!

I never thought for one second the above would become achievable…especially at 50 years old! My below story became my obsession. I set myself a goal. A Black Belt in a Martial Art or nothing! I envisioned the day I earned the highest belt achievable in Martial Arts and made this my goal. I took my eye off the ball towards the end...but I got back on track. We all have goals and dreams and we can all take our eye off the ball (hey, we're human) but only you, can get **YOU** back on track!

So why am I publishing it. I was contacted through a friend to submit my journey to a couple of local newspapers and an online media outlet. 'It can help others' I was told. Decide for yourself. Only YOU can achieve what you set out to do...

Who am I?

As the eldest of four lads growing up in Leeds, England in the seventies and eighties, we enjoyed our childhood. Two hardworking parents ensured we never went hungry and without the necessities. School was one of those parts of your life you have to go through, but I didn't do too bad and had no complaints. I was one of these lads that loved playing soccer. I lived for soccer. Evenings and weekends outside of school and homework would be spent playing soccer under the streetlights, jumpers as goalposts, playing in all weather. I was no superstar, but in my teenage years I enjoyed the training, the soccer matches and then, on reaching that age, the socialising with the lads that came with it. Life was good growing up.

I moved to London, England at the age of twenty-one to earn my millions. My younger brother and cousin lived and worked there and so I was lucky and walked straight into a job and somewhere to live. I didn't earn my millions (nor never believe the person who tells you London's streets are paved with gold!) but I had a fantastic time spending seven years living and working in England's Capital City. I was employed as a drayman, delivering beer to pubs, bars and restaurants, throwing and lifting heavy beer-kegs in and out of cellars, carrying them up flights of stairs, which meant that my fitness levels were never a big concern as my job was now dictating this with so much manual activity. I'd now made several new friends and though we worked hard we also played hard. Saturdays and Sundays were for enjoyment and partying. Weekends back home to Leeds would often mean partying until the last minute and then enduring the seven hour night-bus journey through all the small towns back to London, arriving in Victoria bus-station at 7am just in time for work. No matter how hard you played you made sure work came first (this ethos comes from my upbringing).

I met my wife, Carmel, in London. We worked quite close to each other and her and her friends socialised in the same pub we used as our local. We made the decision to move to Ireland in order to start a family. Three beautiful daughters came along and life was good. We built a house in the country and when we open the blinds are looking out down a valley and river.

I secured manual work, which again, because it was demanding my weight never caused me a second thought. In fact, the work was so demanding I lost three stone (a little below 20 kg's) in a short space of time. Before I knew it and with changes to my work circumstances when the factory relocated abroad, I suddenly found that after all my years of manual work I was now in an office environment which meant I was sitting for long periods of the day.

I NEED TO PUSH MYSELF TO THE LIMITS

Again, life was good living in Ireland and I was approaching my fortieth birthday. My wife and three daughters had planned a surprise party for me. A truly fantastic evening (and weekend!) and it was around this time I decided I wanted to do something that would push me physically, mentally and emotionally, taking me to my limits. I had gotten to an age whereby I noticed my waistline had 'expanded'. Many of us know the feeling. You get the wedding invite, put the suit on you may not have worn in a while and notice the trouser button is under that bit extra pressure. It had to be a long-term challenge and I had to have achieved it by the time I hit mid-century. Ten years to maybe train to swim the English channel or set a goal to run a marathon, something to prove age is only a number. I refuse to be a burden on the health service, being the person with the large stomach hanging over my shorts when on holidays, being unable to tie my shoe-laces, struggling to climb stairs and all those things that can hamper us as we get older. I knew that the next ten years would be my foundations to create a healthier lifestyle for the rest of my life!

A few months had passed when I was laying back in my chair reading a local newspaper. A 'Kickboxing for Beginners' class was starting up near where I work. The organiser was a Martial Arts Black-Belt as well as a two-weight ISKA Kickboxing World-Champion. That was it. It was as if this advert was meant to be seen by me. That was the 'lightbulb' moment. I was going to join a Martial Arts school and go all the way up to Black-Belt. I remember phoning the number on the advertisement, speaking to Tommy McCafferty (Head-Coach and owner of KickboxingLK) and Tommy telling me to come along. That first Tuesday evening walking in and signing up was daunting. I thoroughly understand how difficult it is for anyone taking that first step and why I always help anyone coming along to the club to take that first step. That, in itself, is a huge psychological step with many backing out just before entering through the door.

THAT FIRST STEP...AND TAKING MY EYE OFF THE BALL!

I joined up and was completely bitten by the Martial Arts bug and throughout the early years and I loved it with a passion. Tommy was a twice Kickboxing World-Champion and so I knew I was learning from the best. At the end of a training session I asked how did the grading system work for belts. He told me that grading for belts occurs once per year with a longer period of two years between Brown-Belt and Black-Belt. He said, from his experience, it's a journey of seven or eight years but very few reach the Black-Belt and drop out.   I started my journey and towards the end of my first year I was preparing to grade for my first belt (white). A fantastic feeling to earn my first belt after the hard work I had put in. Preparation for gradings was always intense. I would focus on my training, improving my cardio levels and also using the gym to help my strength and conditioning.   I would drill down on my diet ensuring I was fueling my body with the correct proteins and carbohydrates. The years of grading's was exceptional. The feeling of achievement when reaching each level. It was and has been an amazing journey.

Achieving Brown belt was tough. Mentally, Physically and emotionally tough. I tried not to show it. I was now forty-seven years of age so recovery was taking slightly longer.

Aches and pains seamed to linger that little bit longer but you try not to show it. This was the final belt before achieving Black-Belt. Again, the lead up to grading the training was intensified. Throughout my time I had seen club members being told they weren't up to grading standard and not being allowed to grade. I had seen a number also complete grading, and to be told you need to come back and try again This was not an option in my mind! This, to me would have been a failure. I was so focused and knew I was coming closer to achieving my goal.

I achieved my Brown-Belt and, though I was happy and proud, it wasn't my goal. The last number of weeks had been tough. How would I ever push myself to get that Black belt. I was in the best physical and mental state in my life. I had trained so hard and, without sounding vain, I was forty seven years old and in amazing shape.

I then took my eye off the ball. Took my foot off the gas. Fell off the bandwagon! Call it what you want but I started to get sucked in. I would finish work and go home, making excuses that training was cancelled or I'll get back to it next week. I'd show up for training one night and then miss the next few sessions. I'd build my mind up to get back but then, when the time came I'd think of an excuse! I would pack my training gear and at the last-minute drive past the club. My mind was winning.

Word started to creep out that brown and black-belt grading was coming up in six months. I pulled myself together and got back into training. I trained for one month when, at the end of a session, Tommy asked the club members going for grading to stay behind. I stayed behind also. I asked if I would be grading and was told "No. You won't be grading - sorry Jimmy but you're not training as much as you need to. You're not up to it. Maybe in two years" Tommy said. I was gutted but deep down I knew the answer would be no. Why wouldn't it be! My coach was 100% right. Of course, I didn't see it at the time! I walked out that evening thinking 'I'm through with it'. Time to take the foot off the gas again! I still continued to train but my heart wasn't in it. I didn't want club members to think I was sulking because I had been told 'no'! Then I fell into a decline going from the ultimate of fitness and amazing health into a lazy person with only myself to blame.

I knew through the excuses I was letting my wife and daughters down as they were the ones that questioned why I wasn't training and never once complained throughout the years of Kickboxing (missing school plays, getting home late from training etc.). Why put myself through all that exhaustion when I can go home and open a "few beers" with the feet up munching through crisps, junk food etc. The "few beers" would then be supplemented with a bottle (or two!) of red wine. My fitness levels dropped dramatically. I put on weight (especially around the stomach!) and I even noticed I was taking this lethargic feeling into work. Deep down I was so annoyed with myself. This was Jimmy 90%. Always the 'nearly man' but never finished what he sets out to do! The guys from the club graded for Brown and Black-Belts and I was gutted. Social media lit up with their photos, presentations and messages and I couldn't bring myself to look at it. I couldn't even congratulate them because I was so annoyed with myself!

The company I am employed by provides a yearly checkup of your health. It's a fantastic service whereby a leading health provider send nurses into the workplace to carry out these checks. I had made myself an appointment. I entered the first-aid room and was met by a nurse who, after filling out the required information had my medical history on-hand. This was routine and I knew I had little to worry about. "I'm sorry" said the nurse. "The testing machine appears to be faulty.   Let me get the back-up machine from the car". On testing my blood a second time I was told my cholesterol levels had risen dramatically and that the original test result was correct. "Get to your GP" I was strongly advised "You will be put on a daily tablet for life"...."Oh and by the way, you're also morbidly obese"!

GETTING BACK ON TRACK.

It was around this time of self pity (and cans of beer!) I received a message from the head-coach, Tommy asking was I coming back to training. "You have come so far Jimmy". After exchanging a few messages, I told him I'd be back for the next training session and would get my Black Belt. I made an appointment with my doctor to have my cholesterol levels taken in six weeks' time. This was a sign of an excellent coach. He didn't need to reach out to people. He was running a successful club. But he did and that message was a gesture that helped me re-focus. This was a short-term target to fix what I had broken. Monday morning, I was up early and started training prior to work. I got back into the gym with vengeance prior to Kickboxing training and pushed myself hard. Kickboxing training was excellent and after a few weeks I was, not only back into the swing of things but physically felt better than ever. The buzz returned. Training before work. Gym and Kickboxing training after work. Some evenings back to the gym. I tightened down on my diet. Pasta and chicken all the way. Saturday night was a treat night. Having a treat night was important to me.

Fill the oven with snacks and a few beers and drinks with my family. Heaven! Sunday was getting focused again for the week ahead!

A few weeks in and time to visit my GP. Bloods taken, cholesterol level perfect. Get in there!!

Two years of hard training we were notified that grading for Brown and Black belts was on the horizon and the head-coach, Tommy would be putting forward six club members to grade in Lurgan, Northern Ireland and that other clubs from the north would also be sending members. Would I be one of them? Was I at that level? Had I even trained hard enough? What if I'm told 'no' again? I was in. I was told I would be grading. I was so happy. This was the light at the end of the tunnel. The hard work continued. Kickboxing, gym, Sparring, Early morning training, Cardio sessions, diet, running, alcohol-free. The cycle continued with vengeance! When so many finish their days work on a hot summers evening and sit outside with a cold refreshing drink or winter time when you want to go home and put the feet up in front of the fire with the television on, Not for me! These are the tough times to remain strong and stay focused!

Three months to grading we were told we need to put in extra work as the grading would last six hours. We learnt also that some of these members from other clubs also grading were Irish & UK and European Kickboxing title holders, but this gave us the extra incentive to train harder. Where will I get the time to put in the extra hours of training to last six hours. The answer was simple. I was used getting up early to train before work but now I had to get up at 5am. This was now three months of extra sparring sessions, drilling right down on my diet. My daily intake comprised of pasta, rice, chicken, greens, tuna and water (and plenty of tea). The six of us were held back after putting in tough Kickboxing training sessions and had to complete further fitness drills to push our endurance levels further. I would take myself away from the others and get myself focused. If we were told we had to do an extra one hundred press-ups, sit-ups and burpees I would do two hundred. I would see the others leaving whilst I continued to push myself. No way was I not going to last six hours!

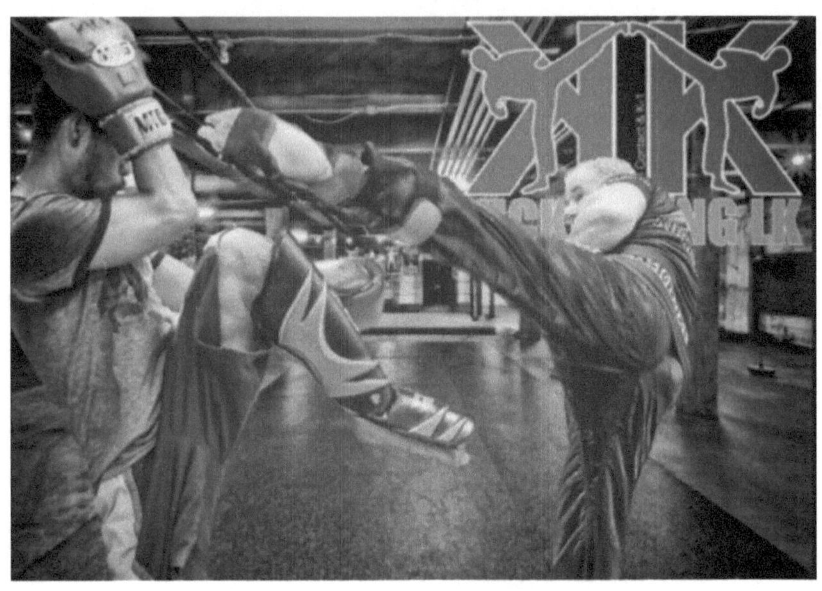

<u>Sparring session</u>

'MEMORABLE' SPARRING SESSION

So, it's the first week of December and the company Christmas dinner-dance. Always an excellent event and always with plenty of alcohol consumed (well it is Christmas!). This year would be different. I was grading the second week in January and I was limiting myself to a glass of wine with dinner. I also had a sparring session the next morning. The good intentions didn't last long. Before you know it, drinks land to the table, it's late into the night, the alcohol is flowing and, when eventually getting a taxi, I crawled into bed at 5am. When the alarm went off early the next morning my head felt as though my brain had exploded. After painfully dragging myself out of bed I made the sixty-kilometer round trip to the club. Tommy seen the sorry state of me walking in and said "Yes Jimmy. You look a bit green. You're sparring with Brian" (Irish Kickboxing champion). After stopping twice to vomit it was a lesson well learned and would never happen again.

GRADING ON THE HORIZON.

Two weeks before grading and, after a training session, Tommy called on of the lads to one side. "Sorry but I can't let you grade. You aren't fit enough". Hearing these words spoken to a club member scared me. It made me train extra hard. I was petrified I might get the same call after a session.

Grading date was the second week in January 2018 so this meant a slightly different Christmas.   I had Christmas Day and New Year's Day off and enjoyed them, but it was then back to training.

Every minute was spent going through combinations in my head. Even when driving I had the combinations playing out loud on my mobile phone. I listened to quite an amount of psychology talks on managing pain.

The week leading up to grading was a week of not sleeping well. Everything was going through my head. Was I fit enough, have I done enough training, where's my gum shield, stay away from anyone with this dreaded flu so I don't catch it! I lay awake at night testing myself on different combinations etc. The first thing I thought of when I woke was combinations! I fell twice when checking my oil tank, both times banging my knee on a rock. I tripped when placing a plate in my dishwasher and a fork went deep under my finger nail causing it to swell and bleed. This can't be happening three days before grading! I had my bag packed two days before grading and kept checking it and re-checking it. I emptied all the contents the night before grading and re-checked them...yet again!

My wife and daughters were amazing. They had stood by me throughout this journey. They had walked with me every step of the way. My wife, Carmel ensured my diet was correct throughout. The conservatory was turned into a gym. My twelve-year-old daughter Katie introduced me into the world of Spotify when out running and the words of encouragement were printed off and placed on the walls. All week I was met with the constant "you can do this" from Carmel and daughters Chloe, Serena and Katie, not forgetting the lovely steak dinner the night before grading. My closest work-colleagues also knew the date and were excellent in support throughout.

Five of us from the club were grading (three going for Brown Belts and two of us going for Black Belt). The last Kickboxing training session, Thursday before grading, our coach, Tommy called us together and told us "That's it. No more training. Take Friday to rest and relax before Saturday". We meet up at the Hotel at 8.30am Saturday morning and travel together.

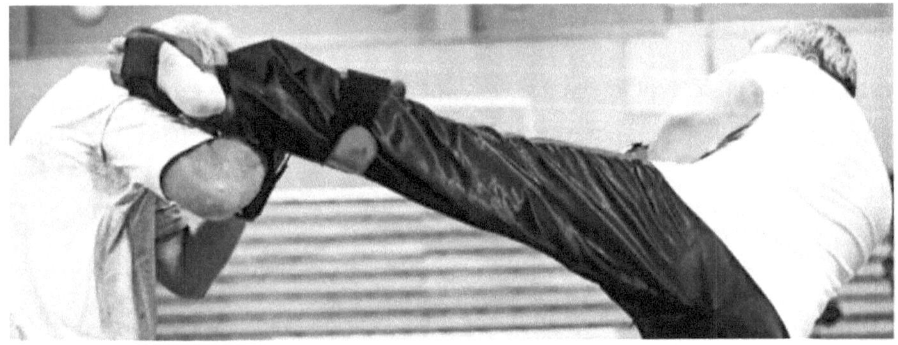

Saturday morning session

GRADING DAY!

Saturday morning, I was buzzing with nervous excitement. My alarm was set for 6.30am. I was up before it sounded. Had I packed everything? If I forget something I won't be allowed to grade. I ate a breakfast of slow-releasing energy food. My wife and daughters were up and having breakfast with me to give me that final bit of encouragement and wave me off. Before I left the house I went to my bedroom, knelt down and said a prayer that I would get through this day. We travelled up to Lurgan in two cars. Tommy kept telling us "no matter how tough it gets, do not give up. You are representing the club and go in with up-most confidence. You are as good as anyone else in there grading today". I couldn't have asked to be heading to Lurgan with a better group of people all willing each other on. My last words to my coach was "Tommy, should I collapse with exhaustion do not let the judges stop my grading. I will get up"!

We arrived at a Martial Arts club I would call 'old-school'. Tough, no airs or graces, a smell of deep-heat hung in the air. It was perfect. Grading was tough and lasted just under six hours. It was outlined to us what was expected during the next six hours and that we would get a break at the half-way point for ten minutes to get fluids into our bodies. If you are not ready to go again at the tenth minute, you're grading is over! If you aren't punching or kicking the Thai pads with all your might, your grading is over! If you are unable to push yourself through the pain barrier of the endurance section, your grading is over! I won't elaborate too much as it wouldn't be fair on others going on to grade but after only fifteen minutes, we were all exhausted wondering how we would last another five hours and forty five minutes. We were soon put at ease when the judge's told us this is nervous exhaustion, and this would pass.

Grading is designed to test your body and mind to its limits as well as techniques, fitness and sparring. I was getting it tough after about four hours when my legs started to cramp. As we continued, the cramps in my legs were showing no mercy and I was getting a stitch from hell

under my ribs.   The heat was unbearable and with the mist in the air and condensation from sweat running down the walls made my throat so sore from thirst. I noticed the condensation running down the walls and at that moment in time would have gladly licked the walls just to get water on my tongue. I had worked on blotting out pain and now was the time to tap into it.

Five hours in and now I had twenty rounds of sparring with different opponents ahead of me. I was completely shot. I had given it my all and was exhausted both mentally and physically. At the seventeenth round of sparring I was digging deep and feeling physically sick and disorientated. This was the part that tested you how much you wanted that Black Belt. The thoughts of that Black Belt and going back to my family spurred me on. Not only that but I was representing the club and I wasn't going back having failed. Between rounds was spent trying to relieve the cramps. Twentieth round and grading was over. I was so exhausted I didn't know if I had done enough. I was annoyed with myself because I felt I had taken kicks and punches I should have defended. I felt my combinations should have been better. Everything ran through my head at that moment for reasons to console myself if I was told 'Sorry – try again in two years'!

We were called together by the judges and congratulated. I was told I had passed the grading. I had done it. In a way I didn't believe it until I seen my name written onto the certificate. I was presented with my Black-Belt by Tommy and he gave me that look and hand-shake to say "you done it". He knew (as did my closest family and friends) what this belt meant to me. Only these people understood the training, the not going out socialising, the salads/pasta nearly every day at work and they were the ones who encouraged me every step of the way!

We stopped off on the journey home to get food (the nicest deep-fried chicken and chips ever) and fluid into us. I went to pay for my food and was told by Tommy "The club pays for this. This is a proud moment".

The drive back home, walking in the door and sharing my moment with Carmel and my daughters had run through my head for years and now it was coming true. I was physically and mentally exhausted, but I was so pumped up with adrenalin. My wife ran me an Epsom salts bath. I seized up and oh-boy did the cramps kick in! That evening and next day was spent resting on the couch and re-hydrating. I lost count of how many times I looked at the belt and certificate over the following weeks and said to myself 'I done it'.

The amount of congratulations and messages I received was amazing but very humbling.

Returning to training on the following Tuesday night was amazing. Two more Black-Belts to add to the club's history. I was still sore, but it was a good pain.

That piece of black cloth you tie around your waist is so important to me. I go through the ritual each and every time I put it on remembering what I had gone through in order to wear it. I explain to others (especially children I now help to coach) the importance of, not only wearing your belt, no matter what colour it is, but the hard work each has put in to earn it...In other words, wear it with pride and honour!

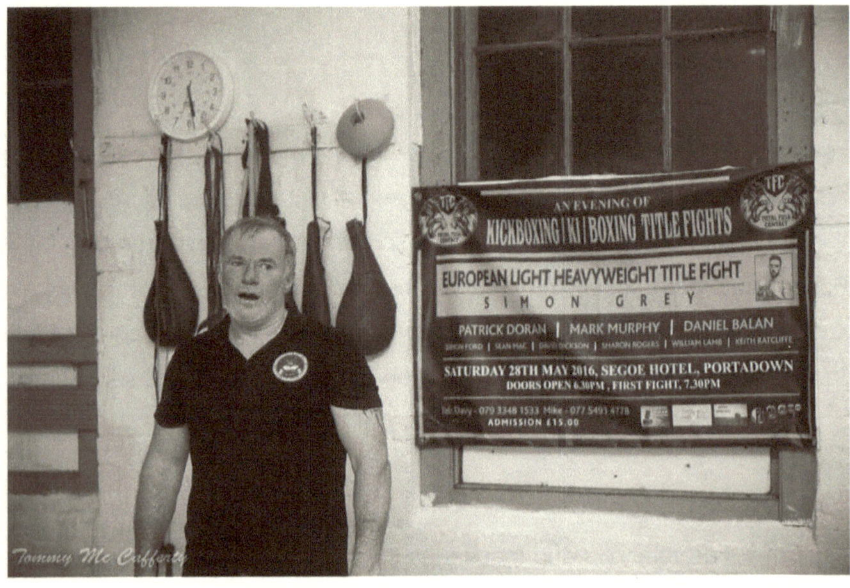

Grading over

IF I CAN SET OUT TO ACHIEVE SOMETHING...SO CAN YOU!

I am so extremely passionate about exercising and the positive effects it has on your body and mind no matter what age you are. It completely changes your outlook on life for the better. I am employed by a large multi-national company. We have a stunning one thousand employee state of the art campus in Ireland. I use the positivity of Martial Arts every day at work to do my very best. I encourage any person that wants to improve their physical fitness and mental wellbeing, to take that first step. I push and promote exercise to others as I know first-hand how it improves both your physical and Mental Health, as well as improving your confidence.

We all have the power within us to motivate but very rarely tap into its full potential. I set a goal. It was just under ten in total to get there. It was tough but it was achievable. Anyone looking to set their own goals, my advice is, take small steps. Set small targets. Reach the targets, applaud yourself (and why not!) and set the next small target.

I achieved my goal in January 2018. In the same year I was honored with three awards for promoting Health and Wellness in the workplace. I hold voluntary morning 'Wake up & Work out' on-site 'boot-camp' style training sessions available to all employees, every morning Monday to Friday (I donate my time for money through the company and donate it to the Mental Health charity 'A Lust for Life'). I not only take the training but also take part. I know first-hand the amazing benefits of exercising prior to starting your days' work, the buzz you get pushing others, the walking out after a training session sweating but the euphoria you feel. If employees want it, the perfect work/wellness opportunity is there. Do your exercising (on-site fitness suite), shower after training (on-site facilities available), head into the work restaurant, grab a free tea/coffee and fruit and then log in, ready to start your days' work!

IS MY JOURNEY OVER? NOT A CHANCE!

Do not tell me you can't !

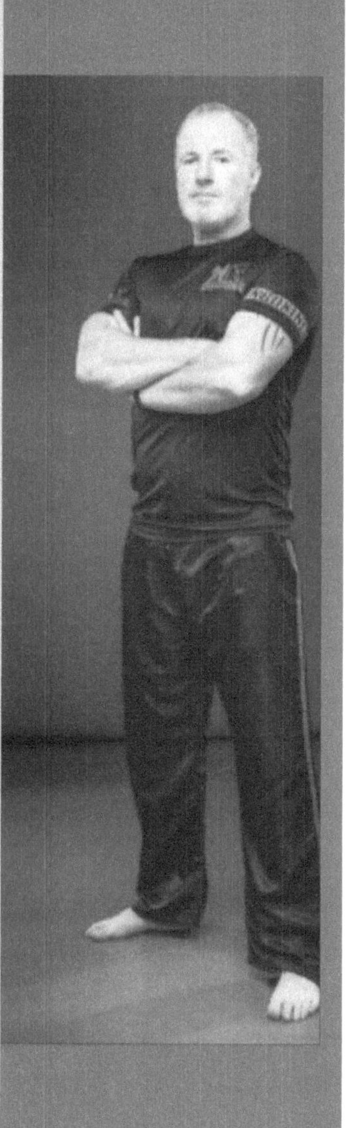

"With the right mindset, positive attitude, and a clear vision of what you want to accomplish, the only thing that is holding you back is yourself".

Apart from the fact achieving my Black-Belt was motivation enough It was a long-term objective that took discipline and vision. I had a target to reach every year (grading for belts) and having this was a massive help to me. Therefore it is so important that if you are setting your own goal you also need to set yourself short-term targets to reach your goal. I talk more about this at the end of my book.

One of my ambitions having reached Black-Belt was to open my own Kickboxing training school and teach but two reasons stopped me.

1: A chance meeting at a training session after reaching my goal.

2: Why open a Kickboxing club when the club I am involved with provides the very best Kickboxing training available, with an excellent history of fighters, Black-Belts and members.

The chance meeting I mention above completely changed my ambitions. Not long after I achieved my Black-Belt, a man (middle-aged, not that this makes a difference) entered the club looking to join up. Throughout the years we have seen many new people come and go so this was nothing out of the ordinary. Tommy, the head-coach asked me if he could train with me and 'show him the ropes'.   My first impressions was this man was confident, had been 'around the block' and could 'look after himself'. He told me he was from Glasgow (a fantastic city but also a city with a tough reputation). After going through a few basics (Kickboxing stance etc.) he started to open up to me as to why he came along to Kickboxing. He told me he had tried to come along twice previously, looked in at the club training and walked away, and became so anxious that it caused him to vomit, on two separate occasions. He didn't mind the physical element (he had boxed when he was younger) but the thoughts of him training in a group made him anxious, thus him vomiting. He told me he had heard about me and my journey and he wanted similar. Wow - was this an eye-opener. I didn't say anything apart from encouraging him and praising him for 'walking through the door' but I took this encounter away with me. There are so many people out there who's Fitness, Health & Wellbeing suffers because they don't have the confidence to exercise in group sessions. It can be such a massive fight with your mind but until this moment it was something I had never noticed previously.

It was after this that I started to pick up more and more how so many people struggle with this (not everybody has the finances to train 1:1 with a personal trainer). This was when I made the decision to change my ambition from opening my own Kickboxing club and go down the road of qualifying as a Fitness Instructor and Personal Trainer. My thought process throughout the years was to open a club and run in in conjunction with Tommy's club but I had noticed the way so many can struggle with their fitness.

Going back to learning in a classroom setting. Similar to the previous ten or eleven years I was the oldest in the class. As you become older it becomes harder for learning to sink in. The physical side of learning was excellent. I was well used to this and could more than hold my own against the younger members. I also had good experience of teaching at both Kickboxing and also providing my own group fitness training sessions. This was a massive benefit to me when it came to the physical training section of the exams. Again, two proud moments for me to achieve certification.

So, where am I at today? The below is not boasting or bragging. It's not about who does Jimmy McCarthy think he is. I'm a humble person. My Kickboxing training teaches respect.

There's also plenty of people out there who have done far more. The below is proof that age should not be used as a factor when it comes to managing your health.

I am fifty two years old. My life has changed since I turned forty. I appreciate and know first-hand the benefits managing your health brings. We all have it within ourselves to be similar so age is not an excuse!

- Black-Belt – Kickboxing.

- Qualified Fitness Instructor & Personal Trainer.

- Twelve years' experience in the Martial Arts & Fitness industry.

- Facilitate Group Fitness / Exercise classes.

- Facilitate 1:1 Fitness training.

- Adults & Children Kickboxing - Back-Belt instructor / Grading examiner.

- Featured on America's largest health insurance company, UnitedHealth Groups 'Stride' Website – Enabling employees to live a healthier lifestyle.

Kickboxing training goes on and will always continue (at least as long as the body allows me). Three times yearly the club run a beginner's class. It's a five-week introduction to Kickboxing and teaches beginners the basics. I step out of my training for the duration to help teach and mentor the new class. Not only is it an opportunity for me to give back to the club but also allows me the chance to go back to basics.

I continue to exercise every morning, Monday to Friday prior to starting my days' work. I train two evenings a week both Gym & Kickboxing (sometimes I might even get a third gym session in). Saturdays it's co-coaching children's Kickboxing and then stay after the class for an hour to do pad-work. Once 6pm on Saturday comes, like I mentioned previously, this is my time to chill out, a few beers, snack food and relax with the family. Training doesn't start again until Monday morning!

Finally – If you are unsure where to start or have a fitness goal you would like to achieve, keep it realistic. Mine was ten years. Yours does not need to be. Start by getting your mind right. Set yourself a starting point and be strict with yourself. Your mind will want to beat you by making every excuse under the sun not to start but don't let it beat you. If you can stay in charge of your mind, you are on the right road to succeeding. Set your goal but include targets that are reachable. Speak to someone who has experienced the change you want to make. Seek advice from a professional who will advise you. When you reach your target reward yourself.

As I say to any member of our club who grade for belts, train hard, if and when you achieve your belt enjoy the moment, get your rest period in and make your very next training session the first session towards achieving your next belt. If you fall off the famous 'band-wagon' look at why you fell off it. Did you lose motivation? Did you not hit the target you had hoped to hit? Did somebody make a comment that knocked your confidence? Don't be critical on yourself! If your goal is to lose weight and tone up, do not become dis-hearted if you put a slight bit of weight on before you start to lose it. This is where so many give up!

Make that change and get back on the 'band-wagon'! When you start to notice change (and if you stick with it, change will come) you will see the amazing lifestyle this change will bring to your life, not just physically and mentally but also to your Health and wellbeing!

'It's not the size of the dog in the fight but the size of the fight in the dog'!

Is my journey over....Not a chance!!

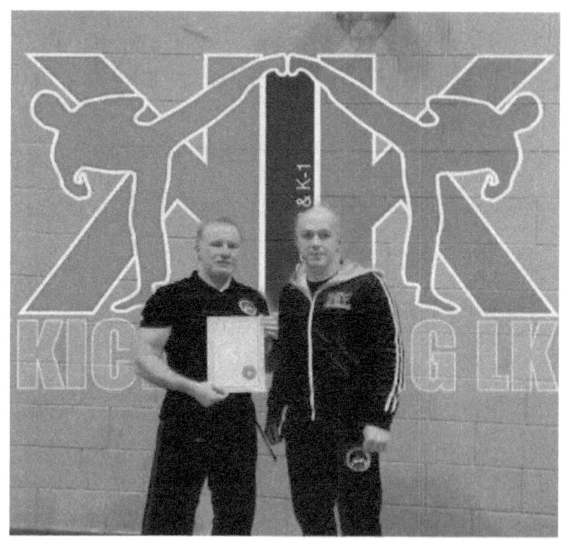

Jimmy McCarthy

Update - Free training programme below

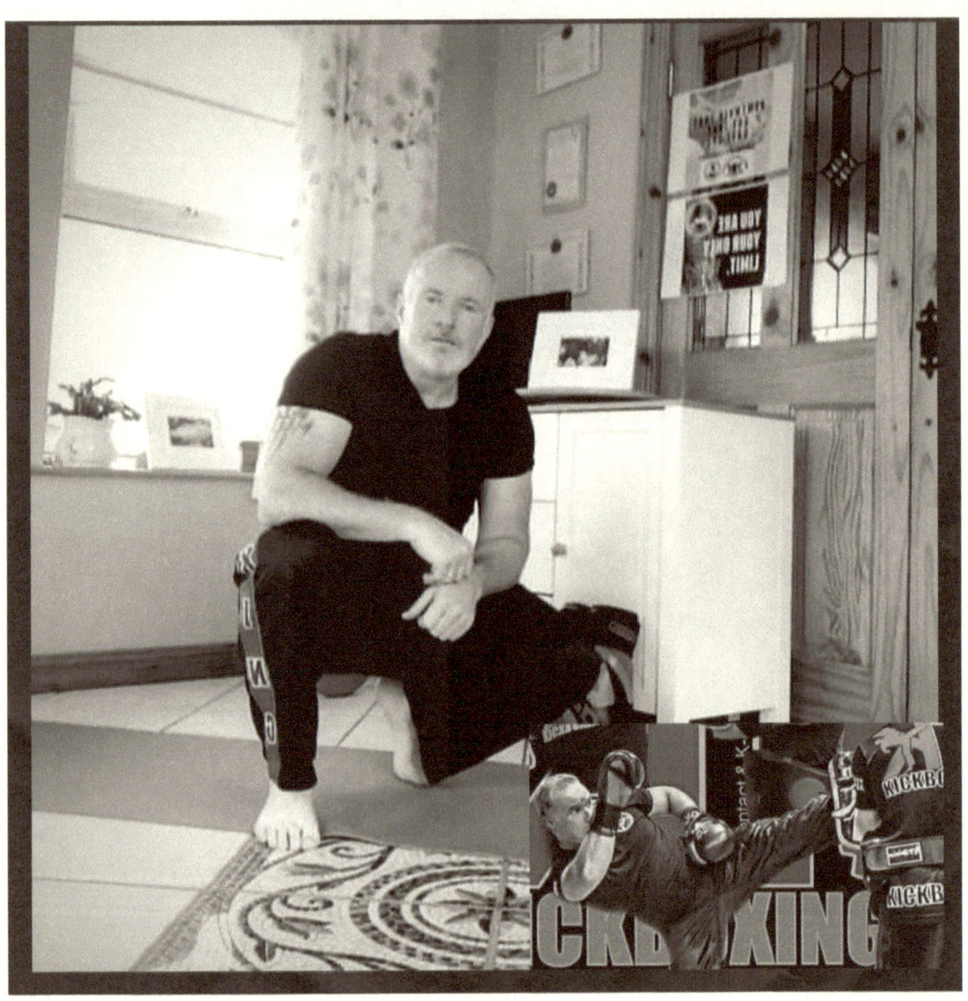
YOU ARE
YOUR ONLY
LIMIT.
KICKBOXING
KICKB

I DIDN'T COME THIS FAR...

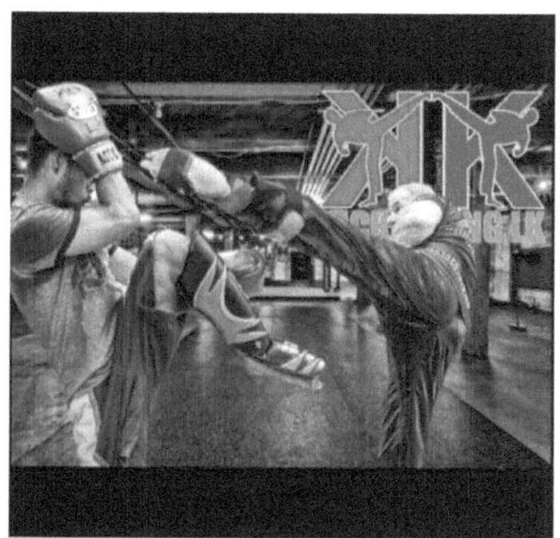

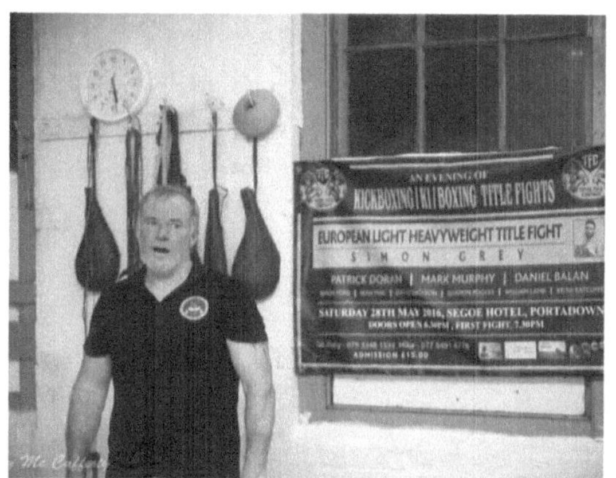

TO ONLY COME THIS FAR!

"All your training isn't doing you much good"

Some people love to throw comments. Use them to your advantage BUT don't go out to prove them wrong. Go out to prove YOU right!

The above quote was said to me one morning. An 'off the cuff' remark said in jest. I laughed it off. Could I have got annoyed? Yes, of course. Did I get annoyed? No. I'm not out to prove anything to other people. My Martial Arts background instills respect. The remark took me by surprise, but I walked away and turned it into a simple positive. I set out to lose 10kg of body fat but with a motive!

If you're one of the countless people that struggle with their weight (and body image) the below just might change your life!

WHO AM I

Before you read any further let me remind you. This section is something I decided to include in a way to help others.

My name is Jimmy McCarthy. I'm just an ordinary person just like you guys. I live in a stunning part of Ireland with my wife, Carmel and three daughters, Chloe, Katie and Serena (oh, and a Jack Russell dog and a cat). When I turned forty years old I set out on a ten year journey, stepping completely outside my comfort zone to achieve a Black-Belt in Kickboxing before I reached the mid-century. It was tough. Very tough! A young persons game? It's mostly younger people take part...but I had a vision...and I achieved it. A massive part of my journey showed me the amazing benefits you receive in life of looking after your health and wellness. This is what I want to share with you.

After reaching my goal I set out to attain my Fitness Instructor and Personal Trainer certification. The past twelve years (I'm now fifty-two years of age) I have learned from the very best. I continue to learn from the very best.

THAT COMMENT

So I've achieved what I set out to achieve. I've learned a hell of a lot. I sacrificed a hell of a lot but my wife and children sacrificed more whilst they stood by me. I still train up to four hours a day outside working full time and family life. I facilitate group fitness training sessions. I work with people who don't have the confidence to exercise in groups. I've spent a lot of time breaking down barriers to give people that skillset to train in group sessions with their head held high.

I was busy holding morning and evening fitness classes and doing all my own training, some days up to four hours a day. I was co-instructing children and teenagers every Saturday at KickboxingLK. A part of my fitness routine also included hitting the weights. I'm around 220lb's (96kg's) and 5ft 9 inches. I went down to 194lb' (88kg's) when I was training for my Black-Belt but after grading I wanted to go back to my 'normal' weight. Let me make it clear, I'm not into body-building where every muscle is defined and diet is extremely strict so I always knew I could lose a bit of body fat if I wanted to, or felt the need.

BECOMING ROUTINE

Exercise is amazing. If done correctly you reap the benefits. If done incorrectly you will have minimal benefit. I took the comment made to me on-board. Yes, on any given day I could be doing five hundred sit-ups. I evaluated and studied my technique and came to the conclusion my exercising had become 'routine'. I looked at my training routine. I drilled down on removing the amount of repetitions I was doing and concentrated on technique and slowing certain exercises down to allow maximum muscle contribution. Instead of doing batches of fifty sit-up's, I honed in on getting the technique right and guess what. I was feeling that good pain from exercising again. I hadn't felt that for a long time as my body had become used to my training. I changed up the combinations to ensure all the correct muscle-groups were being targeted. I designed a short but tough routine. Wow, I was seeing (and feeling results). My stomach started to tone up. Jean's, I had not worn in ten years fitted me again.

SUPER SPIRULINA

It was also around the same time I had heard about a relatively unknown super-food called Spirulina and started to research its benefits. I found out that this pond-life alga was used in Japanese diets. The Japanese are smart people so why were they using this in their diet? Spirulina, when ingested helps to remove the visceral (bad) fats from your body. The fats that build up, in particular, around your vital organs located in your body's midriff, the belly and the famous 'love-handles', to put it bluntly. It is quite possibly the most under-rated super-food out there but so very unknown.

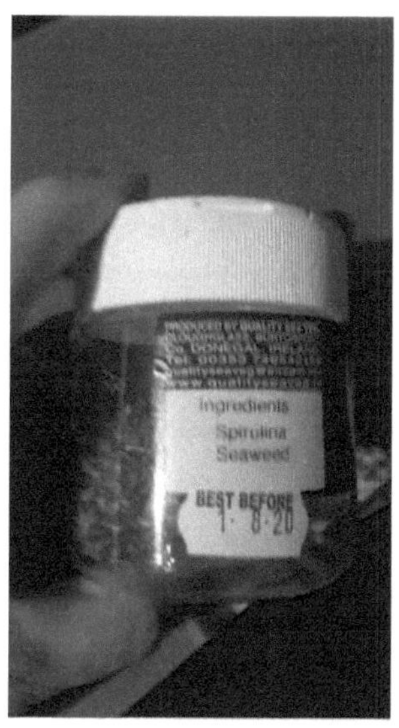

Spirulina

As I mentioned, Spirulina is still a relatively unknown product. Though becoming more available to buy off the shelf it hardly moves from the shelves of supermarkets or health-food stores because so few people are aware of it's amazing properties. I facilitate so much fitness and exercise teaching with others but I had an idea for a future fitness drive. The comment made to me wasn't far off the mark. I had around twenty-two pounds (ten Kilograms) of body fat I could lose. I set myself a six-week program to introduce Spirulina into my diet, combined with an exercise session to target the mid-section of the body (around the belly). My routine was simple. It didn't consume every minute of my being. Let me tell you this though and I apologies if this is uncomfortable. When you first introduce Spirulina into your diet, it is unforgiving! When you use the toilet..well, let's just say it heightens the sense of smell. Put it another way, your body waste stinks!! If you're taking Spirulina as part of an exercise plan you are also breaking down stubborn body fat that may have been inside your body for a long time. When it comes out it stinks!! Not nice I know but it is what it is. I stepped on the weighing scales and was down to 189lb's (86kg's). The program is below. The food I made is also below. I have even included a link to my exercise routine to exercise and stretch the mid-section of the body. It was a win-win. I lost the weight in four weeks!

I PUT MY MONEY WHERE MY MOUTH IS!

The routine had worked.   I hadn't consumed every waking hour battling to get my weight down. Once I had set out to reach this weight, I was going to put the weight back on in a clean way. More importantly was I was going to promote classes using this super-food alongside the exercise routine I had devised. Some people like to diet but don't like to exercise. Others like to exercise but don't want to lose weight, i.e. muscle-mass. This class was specifically designed for any person looking to reduce body fat. The feedback spoke for itself. Participants joined in and followed my plan. They continued this over a six week span. The only reason for taking two weeks more than me was because I had to spend the first two weeks getting them past the pains of first exercising.

CONCLUSION

When it comes to paying money to improve your fitness and health then you want results! You've spent your hard-earned money and invested your trust with somebody, so I want you to get results. Follow the below for six weeks. Follow the program Monday to Friday. Allow yourself the weekend (or two days together) if you work weekends. This is important for two reasons:

1. Allows your body to rest and repair.
2. Allow yourself a weekend treat. You've worked hard all week so why not have a Saturday night to yourself! Just remember though, you cannot burn off a bad diet if you go overboard!

The plan you should follow is below but feel free to change the food I prepared (Fritata), or add Spirulina to food you enjoy (sensible foods)!

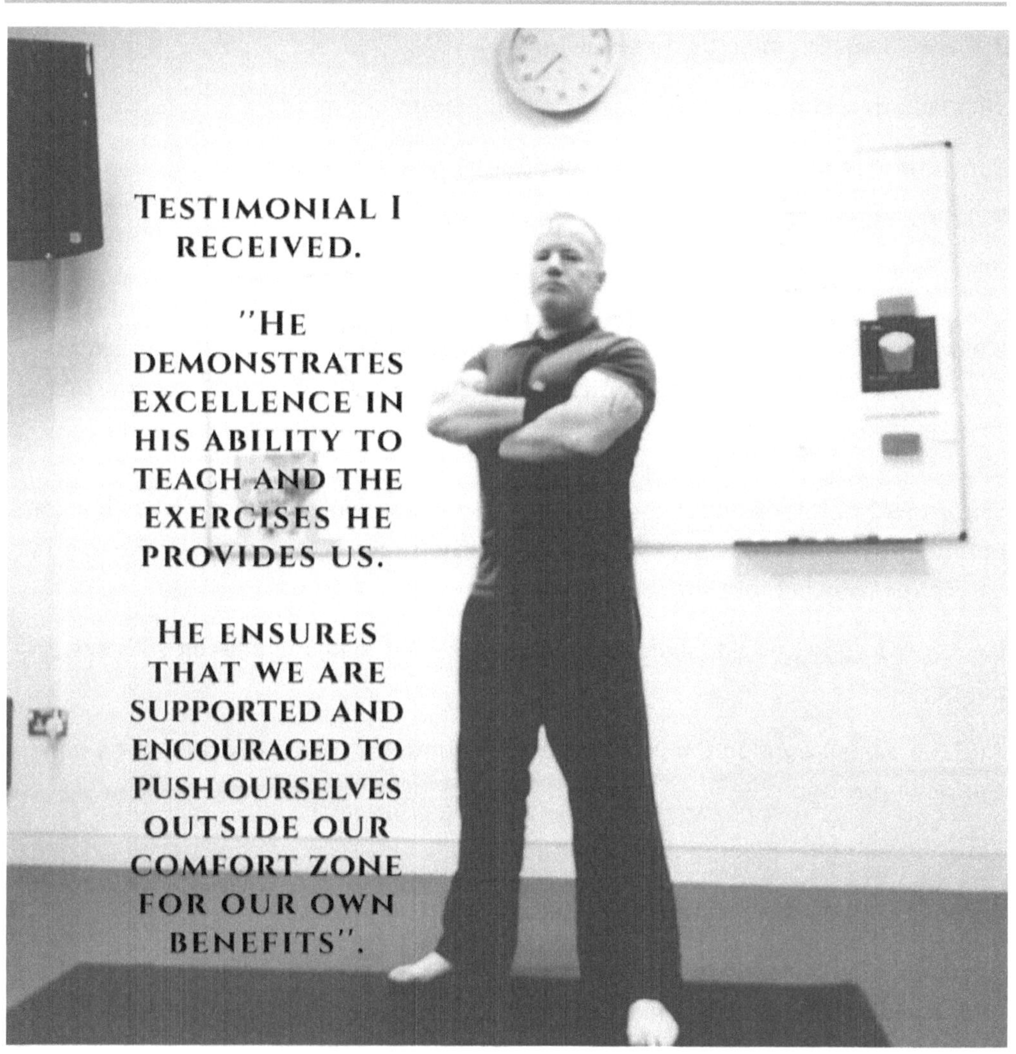

Monday - Friday

7:30am - 8am. Exercise using the below link.

10:30am. Breakfast. A bowl of natural yogurt with chopped fruit.

1pm. Lunch. Fritata with Spirulina (contents below).

5pm. Chicken and vegetables (or pasta).

Making your Fritata. I make mine every evening for the following day to eat at work. It takes fifteen minutes to make and so simple. I eat it cold. It's amazing.

Chop 1 to 2 potatoes (leave the skin on. This is amazing fiber) and fry in a small amount (two tablespoons) of vegetable oil. Fry for ten minutes. Feel free to add carrots/pees/sweetcorn/broccoli etc.

Beat 2 or 3 eggs and add a small amount of low-fat milk and season with salt and pepper.

Add the beaten eggs to the potatoes and continue to cook. Add 1 teaspoon of Spirulina powder.

Finish cooking by placing the pan under a grill.

Allow to cool before placing into a lunchbox and refrigerating.

Every evening before bed make a cup of Ginger tea or Green tea with a teaspoon of Spirulina stirred through (add honey if it's tough to take). This is in your body nicely working away whilst you sleep.

Follow this link to my YouTube class. It's an eight-minute workout focused on your abdominal muscles and obliques. We all have them. Sometimes we need to work them:

https://youtu.be/Tb3cqoS98UI (if the link does not work type into the search-box 'PecsFactor').

Take part in the online class once a day Monday to Friday. Ensure you are in good medical condition. If unsure you should seek medical advice from your doctor. Ensure you have water.

You will start to notice a difference. When you receive compliments take them with both hands! Why wouldn't you accept the compliments. You've worked damn hard for what you have achieved!

Thank you and good luck.

Jimmy

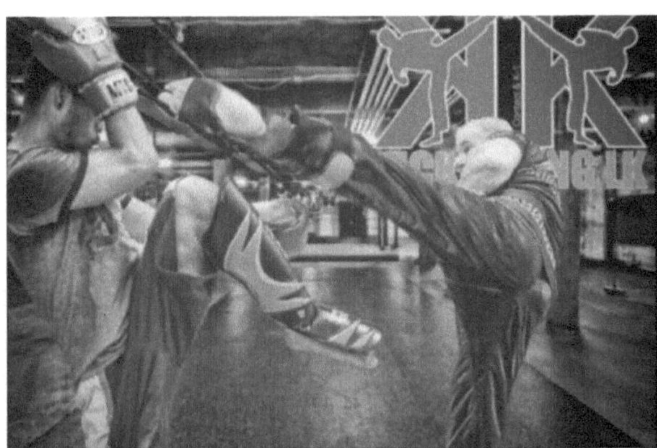

PECSFACTOR.COM
Kickboxing Black-Belt
Qualified Fitness Instructor
Qualified Personal Trainer